**W9-DBH-310**

# TOO MANY SUNDAY DINNERS

## FAMILY AND DIET

# OBESITY & KIDS

# TOO MANY SUNDAY DINNERS

## FAMILY AND DIET

### BY RAE SIMONS

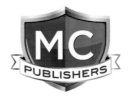

Mason Crest Publishers

MASON CREST PUBLISHERS INC.
370 Reed Road
Broomall, Pennsylvania 19008
(866)MCP-BOOK (toll free)
www.masoncrest.com

First Printing
9 8 7 6 5 4 3 2 1

Library of Congress Cataloging-in-Publication Data

Simons, Rae, 1957–
  Too many Sunday dinners : family and diet / by Rae Simons.
    p. cm. — (Obesity & kids)
  Includes bibliographical references and index.
  ISBN 978-1-4222-1713-9 (hardcover)    ISBN 978-1-4222-1705-4 (hardcover series)
  ISBN 978-1-4222-1901-0 (pbk.)        ISBN 978-1-4222-1893-8 (pbk series)
  1. Obesity—Juvenile literature. 2. Obesity—Genetic aspects—Juvenile literature. I. Title.
  RC628.S622 2010
  616.3'98—dc22
                        2010019188

Design by Wendy Arakawa.
Produced by Harding House Publishing Service, Inc.
www.hardinghousepages.com
Cover design by Torque Advertising Design.
Printed in the U.S.A. by Bang Printing.

The creators of this book have made every effort to provide accurate information, but it should not be used as a substitute for the help and services of trained professionals.

# CONTENTS

# INTRODUCTION
## FOR THE TEACHERS

We as a society often reserve our harshest criticism for those conditions we understand the least. Such is the case for obesity. Obesity is a chronic and often-fatal disease that accounts for 400,000 deaths each year. It is second only to smoking as a cause of premature death in the United States. People suffering from obesity need understanding, support, and medical assistance. Yet what they often receive is scorn.

Today, children are the fastest growing segment of the obese population in the United States. This constitutes a public health crisis of enormous proportions. Living with childhood obesity affects self-esteem, which down the road can affect employment and attainment of higher education. But childhood obesity is much more than a social stigma. It has serious health consequences.

Childhood obesity increases the risk for poor health in adulthood—but also even during childhood. Depression, diabetes, asthma, gallstones, orthopedic diseases, and other obesity-related conditions are all on the rise in children. Recent estimates suggest that 30 to 50 percent of children born in 2000 will develop type 2 diabetes mellitus, a leading cause of preventable blindness, kidney failure, heart disease, stroke, and amputations. Obesity is undoubtedly the most pressing nutritional disorder among young people today.

If we are to reverse obesity's current trend, there must be family, community, and national objectives promoting healthy eating and exercise. As a nation, we must demand broad-based public-health initiatives to limit TV watching, curtail junk food advertising toward children, and promote physical activity. More than rhetoric, these need to be our rallying cry. Anything short of this will eventually fail, and within our lifetime obesity will become the leading cause of death in the United States if not in the world. This series is an excellent first step in battling the obesity crisis by educating young children about the risks, the realities, and what they can do to build healthy lifestyles right now.

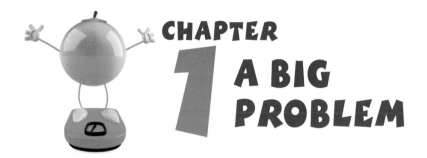

# CHAPTER 1

# A BIG PROBLEM

Did you know that people all over the globe are getting fatter? There are more than 1 billion adults around the world who are **overweight**. At least 300 million of them are **obese**.

But it's not just grownups who are overweight and obese. More and more children are overweight too, even very young children. Around the world, at least 42 million children who are younger than five are overweight.

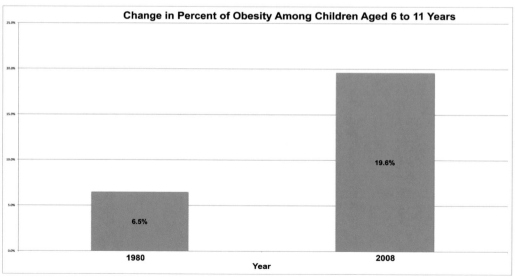

*This chart shows how childhood obesity has increased in the United States from 1980 to 2008. Obese children are more likely to become obese or overweight adults.*

# HOW DO YOU KNOW IF YOU'RE OVERWEIGHT?

Experts have figured out a way to help you know if you are in the healthy weight range for your height. It's called the body mass index or BMI. The BMI formula uses height and weight to come up with a BMI number. Though the formula is the same for adults and children, figuring out what the BMI number means is a little more complicated for kids. For children, BMI is plotted on a growth chart that tells whether a child is underweight, healthy weight, overweight, or obese. Different BMI charts are used for boys and girls who are younger than twenty, because the amount of body fat differs between boys and girls. Also, the amount of body fat that is healthy is different, depending on whether you're a toddler or a teenager.

**What's the difference between being overweight and being obese?** Both words mean that a person has too much body fat, so much so that it's a health risk. But a person who is obese has much more fat than a person who is overweight, and the health risks are greater as well.

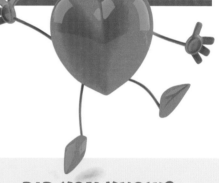

## DID YOU KNOW?

Most very healthy individuals have less than 15 percent body fat. In other words, at least 85 percent of their total body weight is made up of non-fat cells.

## 2 to 20 years: Boys
## Body mass index-for-age percentiles

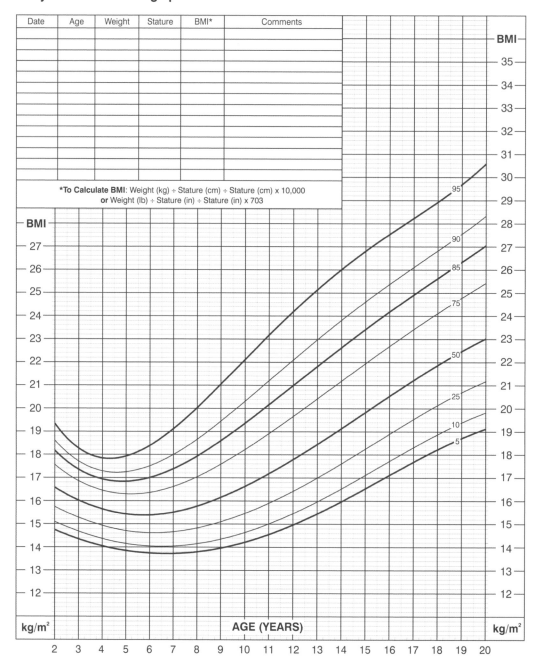

| Date | Age | Weight | Stature | BMI* | Comments |
|------|-----|--------|---------|------|----------|
| | | | | | |

*To Calculate BMI: Weight (kg) ÷ Stature (cm) ÷ Stature (cm) x 10,000
or Weight (lb) ÷ Stature (in) ÷ Stature (in) x 703

*BMI growth chart for boys ages 2–20.*

**2 to 20 years: Girls**
**Body mass index-for-age percentiles**

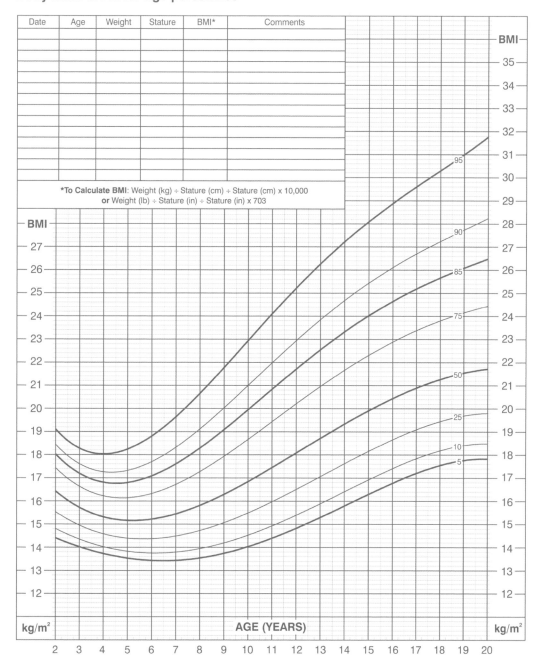

*BMI growth chart for girls ages 2–20.*

Each BMI chart is divided into percentiles. A child whose BMI is equal to or greater than the 5th percentile and less than the 85th percentile is considered a healthy weight for his or her age. A child at or above the 85th percentile but less than the 95th percentile for age is considered overweight. A child at or above the 95th percentile is considered obese. A child below the 5th percentile is considered underweight.

If you know how much you weigh and how tall you are, you can look at these charts and see for yourself whether you are overweight or obese—but it's also a good idea to talk to your doctor (even if that seems embarrassing). BMI is not always right, so a doctor will be better able to tell you if your weight is healthy or not.

## DID YOU KNOW?

In the United States, 15 percent of all children between the ages of 6 and 11 are overweight. That means that if you have 100 children in a room, chances are 15 of them would be overweight. Next, if you were to put 100 kids who were between the ages of 12 and 19 all in one room, you'd be likely to find that 18 of them (18 percent) would be overweight. And if you then put 100 grownups together, 67 of them would be overweight or obese. That's more than two-thirds of all grownups!

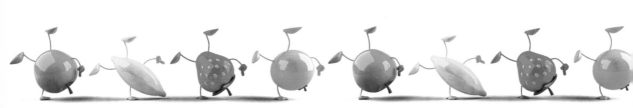

# THE DANGERS OF BEING OBESE OR OVERWEIGHT

Being overweight or obese isn't healthy. It puts you at risk for getting sick, both now, when you're still a kid, and later, when you grow up. It's a big problem!

Children who are overweight or obese are more likely to get diabetes. This is a disease where your body doesn't break down sugar the way it should. If you have diabetes, you will probably have to take medicine or have special shots every day to help your body process sugar normally. Diabetes can lead to other diseases as well, including blindness. It can make it hard for you to heal after a cut or injury.

Being overweight also increases your chances of having heart disease. This is an illness we usually connect with older people, but carrying too much weight

## DID YOU KNOW?

The term doctors and scientist use for fat is adipose tissue. It's made up of special cells that store lipids. Lipids are packed with energy, so adipose tissue is a good way for your body to store energy that you'll need later on. Your body's energy comes from the food you eat. When you eat more food than you need to meet your daily energy needs, your body changes the extra energy into lipids, which are stored as adipose tissue—or fat. This is a good thing, because it means your body can keep going even if it has to go without food for a while. But when you have more adipose tissue—more fat—than your body can use, it can be dangerous to your health.

around is hard on your heart, no matter how old you are. Even worse, the heavier you are, the harder it will probably be for you to run around and exercise. Your heart and lungs need exercise to be healthy. Today, more and more children are obese or overweight—and more and more children are getting heart disease.

Overweight children are also likely to stay that way as they grow up. Being obese or overweight when you are an adult can put you at risk for even more diseases. The extra weight puts strain on your joints, which can lead to arthritis, a disease that makes your joints swollen, stiff, and sore. Obesity may also cause certain kinds of **cancer**.

As people who are overweight or obese grow older, the added weight on their bodies can also lead to other problems, like **high blood pressure** (which increases your chances of having a **stroke**),

**What is cancer?** Cancer is a disease that causes the cells in different parts of your body to grow too fast, to the point that they kill healthy cells.

**What do high blood pressure and stroke mean?** High blood pressure is when blood pushes against the walls of the blood vessels harder than is normal. This tends to happen when the vessels become too narrow.

A stroke is when the cells in your brain suddenly die because they don't get enough blood.

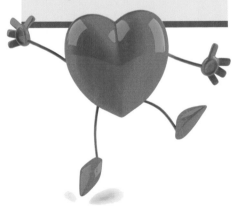

**What is your gallblad-
der?** Your gallbladder
is an organ in your body
that helps you digest fats.

**What is depression?**
Depression is an
emotional illness that
makes people feel very
sad most of the time.

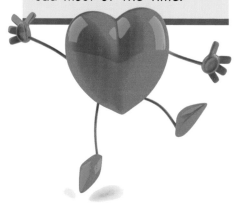

## DID YOU KNOW?

Even though doctors use BMI to
determine if you're overweight or
obese, BMI is sometimes wrong. That's
because different types of body
tissues weigh different amounts.
Muscle, for example, weighs eight
or nine times as much as fat. This
means that a small amount of muscle
will be as heavy, or heavier, than
a larger amount of fat.

Imagine two children who
are the same height. One weighs
100 pounds. The other weighs
85 pounds. Judging by weight
alone, you might think that the
85-pound child is healthier and has
less fat than the 100-pound child.
If the 100-pound kid, however,
is very muscular, and the 85-pound
kid has practically no muscles
at all, then you'd be wrong. The
85-pound child could actually
be both lighter and "fatter" than
the muscular 100-pound kid.

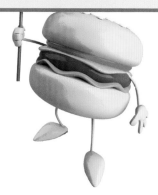

**gallbladder** disease, and
breathing problems. Being
overweight can also mean
that you have more prob-
lems handling your emo-
tions. People who are obese
or overweight are more likely
to have **depression**.

## A COMPLICATED PROBLEM

Our world is full of messages telling us we need to be thin to be pretty or good-looking. Everywhere we turn—on television, in ads, on magazine covers—we run into this message. Every year, thousands and thousands of people—including kids—go on diets. They buy exercise equipment and join gyms. They drink diet sodas and eat special low-fat foods. And yet people around the world are still getting fatter.

Not everyone understands that obesity is a health problem rather than an appearance problem. Sometimes people think that others who are overweight are lazy or greedy. They think that if those people wanted to lose weight bad enough, they could easily become thinner. Sometimes people don't want to get to know others simply because they're overweight or obese. They assume that people with more fat are not as interesting, not as smart, or simply not as important.

### DID YOU KNOW?

In the United States, 15 percent of all children between the ages of 6 and 11 are overweight. That means that if you have 100 children in a room, chances are 15 of them would be overweight. Next, if you were to put 100 kids who were between the ages of 12 and 19 all in one room, you'd be likely to find that 18 of them (18 percent) would be overweight. And if you then put 100 grown-ups together, 67 of them would be overweight or obese. That's more than two-thirds of all grownups!

Prejudice is the word we use when we think differently about others because of their race, their religion, or the way they look. Most of us know that this is wrong—but many people think it's okay to think about people differently because they are overweight or obese. This is a form of prejudice too. And yet we hear fat jokes at school all the time. Grownups tell fat jokes too. People on television do as well. Most of the time, people forget how cruel this is, or how it makes others feel.

People come in all different sizes and shapes— and no one should ever be insulted or treated with less respect because of their weight. People who are overweight or obese can still be smart and pretty and funny. And losing weight isn't easy.

Obesity is a complicated problem. Eating and exercise habits are a big part of the problem, but it's not always that simple. Your weight is also shaped by the family you were born into. The way your body is made and the way you live your life depends partly on the traits your parents passed along to you—and they in turn had **traits** passed on to them by *their* parents. It's a process that scientists call "heredity." And it's very hard to change these earliest, most basic **influences**!

**DID YOU KNOW?**

Being overweight and not exercising enough causes one-third of all cancers.

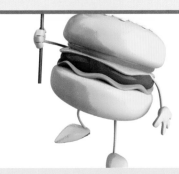

**What are traits?** They are the characteristics you have. They include things like the color of your hair and how tall you are, as well as things like your talents, your personality, and the way your body handles the food you eat.

**What are influences?** They're things that shape you to be one thing or another. Influences don't MAKE you be a certain way—but they give you a push in that direction.

**DID YOU KNOW?**

We often think of pigs and fatness together. But pigs are also the victims of untrue stereotypes. In reality, pigs are not normally fat. If they have their choice, they are not normally dirty (they do like to roll in mud on hot, sunny days, but that's only because they get sunburned easily). And pigs are very intelligent.

So remember: stereo-types are often simply not true!

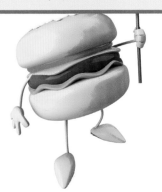

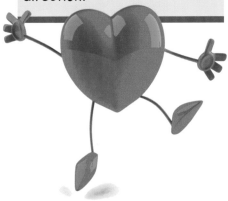

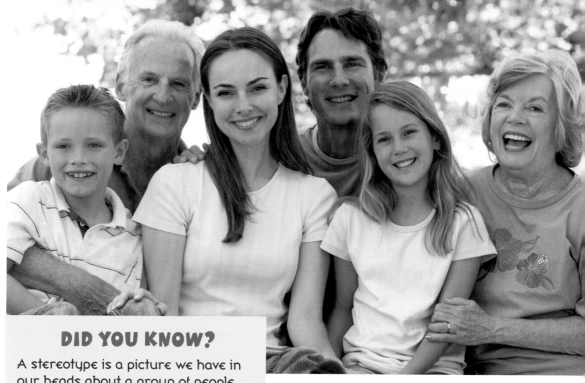

## DID YOU KNOW?

A stereotype is a picture we have in our heads about a group of people. It's not necessarily true. In fact, it seldom is, because people are individuals, and each person within a group is different. But many people have a stereotype in their heads when they think about people who are overweight and obese. They think that they're lazy, weak, and sad. They may think people who are overweight are not as clean or that they smell bad. They often think people who are overweight and obese are not as smart and not as likeable as other people.

And that's not true.

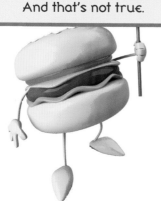

*The family you grow up with shapes your life—you inherit traits from your grandparents and parents that make you look a certain way. In addition, your family teaches you ideas and habits that help make you into the person you are.*

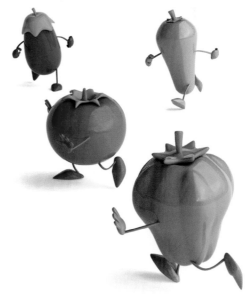

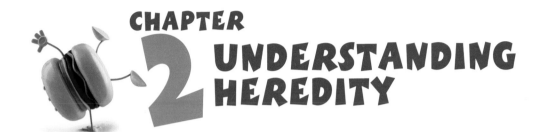

# CHAPTER 2 UNDERSTANDING HEREDITY

Heredity has to do with inheriting things—in other words, when something is handed down from one generation to another. For instance, you might inherit your grandmother's jewelry. Or one day, when your parents die, you might inherit their house or their other belongings.

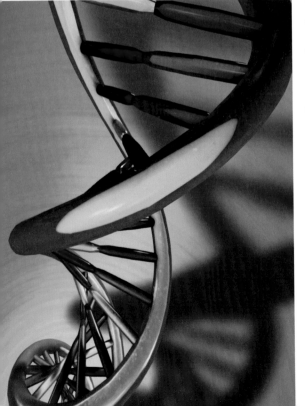

*DNA, the chemical that tells your cells what to become, is shaped like a twisted ladder.*

When scientists talk about heredity, though, they usually mean the physical traits we inherit from our parents. If your parents are tall, for example, chances are good you'll be tall too. You might inherit your mom's blue eyes or your dad's curly hair. You can also inherit things that aren't as easy to see, like intelligence or stubbornness or musical talent. These things are passed down to you through your parents' genes.

# WHAT ARE GENES?

All the information for what your body looks like is stored within each cell of your body, on a tiny corkscrew-shaped chemical called DNA. DNA is like a map that tells all your cells what to become—and it was passed along to you from your parents. Every cell in your body has a complete copy of the DNA you got from each of your parents.

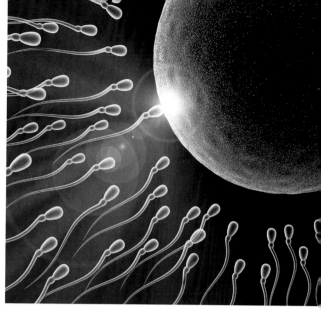

*One of your father's sperm cells joined with your mother's egg cell to make you. Many other sperm cells tried, but only one was successful—if a different one had joined with the egg, you'd be a different person!*

DNA's spiral is made of genes. Genes in turn are organized into long strands called chromosomes. Human beings have 46 chromosomes, which come in 23 pairs. Half of the chromosomes comes from your mother. The other half comes from your father.

# HOW DO GENES WORK?

Your DNA was formed at the moment you were conceived—the moment when your father's sperm cell came together with your mother's egg cell. Unlike all the other cells in the human body, egg and sperm cells don't have pairs of chromosomes. Instead, they have only half the double strand that all the other cells have. So when an egg cell and a sperm cell meet, the 23 chromosomes in each of them join together—and create a completely new cell with 46 chromosomes. This new cell has its own brand-new DNA map—and it uses that map to copy itself over and over, until an entirely new human being grows from it, a person who will have traits from both parents.

Scientists have learned that some genes are stronger than others. For example, the gene for brown eyes is stronger than the gene for blue eyes. Scientists call the stronger gene the "dominant" gene and the weaker one the "recessive" gene. This means that if you inherit from your mother the gene for blue eyes, while your father passes along the gene for brown eyes, your eyes will probably be brown, because brown is the dominant, or stronger, gene.

Sometimes, though, more than one gene shapes the same quality. Scientists have discov-

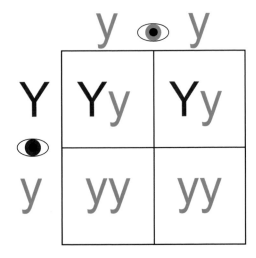

This Punnett square shows how dominant genes and recessive genes work to make traits. The trait for brown eyes "Y" is dominant over the trait for green eyes "y"—a person only needs one "Y" to have brown eyes, but must have two "y"s to have green eyes.

ered this is actually true for eye color. That's why there are so many different shades of eye color, from brown to hazel to green to blue, with lots of variations of each one.

Genes are complicated. Scientists didn't even know they existed until the 1950s, and today they're still learning more about them. For those of us who aren't scientists, genes are even harder to understand.

Some traits we inherit from our parents are clear cut and definite. Your eyes are either blue or brown (or something in between). Your hair is either straight or curly—either blonde, brown, or red. But other things aren't as definite. For instance, if your mother is a famous artist, you might inherit some of her talent—but you won't automatically be a famous artist too. You might choose to do something very different with your life, like become a lawyer or a farmer or an athlete. You might never develop the talent you inherited from your mother.

**What's environment mean?** The environment is everything around you—the community where you live, your family, your house, your school.

Many other traits we inherit from our parents will also be shaped by the things around us as we grow up. It's a complicated mixture of genes, **environment**, and our individual choices.

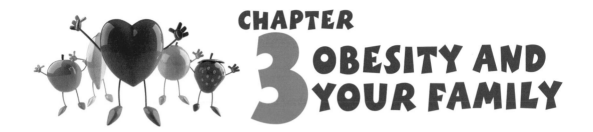

If you have a sore throat that doesn't go away, your mom or dad will probably take you to the doctor. If you had a more serious illness, like cancer, for example, you would spend a lot of time being treated by doctors whose jobs would be to help you recover from your disease. But if you're overweight, you may not think of yourself as needing help from a doctor. You probably don't look at obese people and think, "They have an illness."

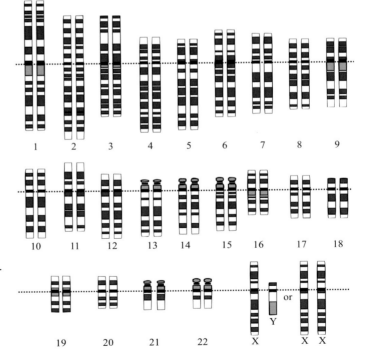

*This image, called a karyotype, is a map of the 23 pairs of chromosomes in your cells.*

But today, most doctors and scientists agree that obesity is a disease. It's not just a question of a person making bad choices about diet and exercise. Of course poor eating habits and lack of exercise play important roles in obesity, but they're not the whole story by any means. **Researchers** today agree that being obese or overweight is also connected to your family. If your parents and grandparents were overweight, you're not doomed to be overweight too—but the chances are much higher that you will be.

**What are researchers?** They're people who study things and try to discover the answers to questions.

There are two reasons for this. One has to do with your genes—and the other has to do with your family's lifestyle.

# GENES AND OBESITY

Scientists today are trying to create a map that tells what each gene controls. They already know what some of the genes do. For example, they know which genes make you a boy or a girl. They know which genes control certain diseases. But there are many, many genes that scientists still haven't put on their map. What makes the process even harder and more complicated is that many illness-es and conditions are controlled by more than one gene.

Scientists have, however, found a few single-gene conditions that can cause obesity. One of these genes has to do with how your body produces a chemical called leptin.

Leptin has an important job in your body. It tells your body how much food it needs and how much energy to use. Fatty tissue makes leptin, so the more fat you have, the more leptin your body makes. Special **sensors** in your brain can tell how much leptin you have flow-ing in your blood, and if they see that there's a lot of leptin, they make your body feel less hungry. If they sense less leptin in your blood, they make you feel hungrier. That's how it's supposed to work anyway.

**What are sensors?**
They're things—either ma-chines or, as in this case, parts of the body—that react to sounds, light, heat, or certain chemicals (for example) in a certain way, with a specific reaction.

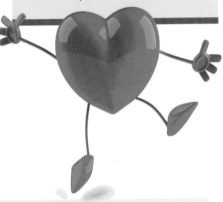

## DID YOU KNOW?

Human DNA contains so much in-formation that if you were to write it down in book form, you would need 200 volumes the size of a Manhattan telephone book (1,000 pages each)! If you were going to try to read it out loud to someone, you would need nine and a half years to get through the entire "story" (without stopping).

**DID YOU KNOW?**

Each person has about one billion different genes! Scientists think that about 25,000 to 35,000 of these are important to each individual's unique identity.

So the more fat you have, the less hungry you should feel. But for some people, that's not how their bodies work. Instead, the sensors in their brains can't tell how much leptin they have—so they never turn off their hunger. The people who have the gene that controls this condition will feel hungry all the time. No matter how much they eat, they still feel hungry. For these people, it's not a question of not having any will power. When you feel like you're starving all the time, it's pretty hard to control your eating habits!

Scientists have discovered that they can turn on the leptin sensors in these people's brains. When they do, these people can suddenly lose weight. Within just a year, they're no longer obese

*A chromosome carries genes, which in turn are made up of DNA.*

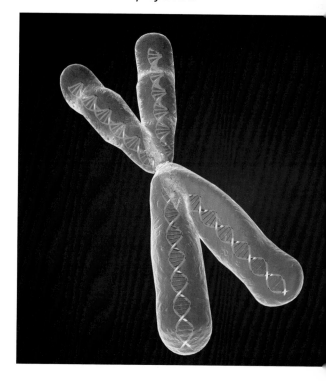

or overweight. For people like this, medical treatment must seem like a miracle.

Other genes can cause similar conditions, making people hungry all the time, Other genes get in the way of the body using energy, so that instead of "burning" calories, it keeps on storing fat. Researchers are finding the answers to some of these problems, and their answers offer health and hope to people who are overweight or obese.

Certain genes can cause special problems like these in some people—but other genes may be more common. Scientists believe that in the past our ancestors needed to develop the genes that would allow them to keep eating despite no longer being hungry. These genes were useful because human beings had to survive periods when food was less common. When

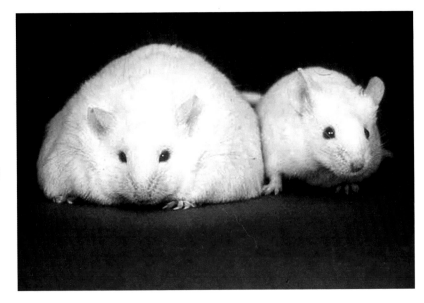

Scientists found that mice without the leptin gene become obese, just like people without the gene.

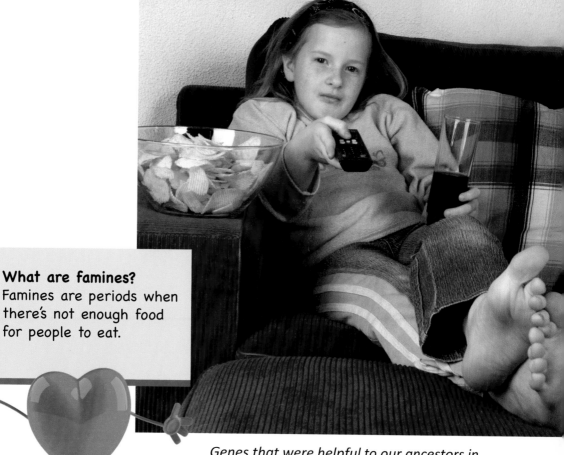

**What are famines?**
Famines are periods when there's not enough food for people to eat.

*Genes that were helpful to our ancestors in times of famine are now telling us to eat even when we don't need to. Many of us snack without thinking—eating in front of the T.V. is a good example of unnecessary eating.*

they had plenty of food to eat, their bodies needed to be able to take in lots of energy and then store it in the form of fat that would get them through **famines**.

The people who had these genes were able to survive long, cold winters and hot, dry summers—and this meant they lived to pass along their genes to their children, who in turn passed the genes along to THEIR children, and so on, down the long chain of the **generations** until today.

And now many of us still have the genes that tell our bodies to keep eating even when we're no longer truly hungry. The problem is, however, most of us no longer have to survive without food for long periods of time. But we still eat, even when we don't really need to. We may eat when we're bored or sad or lonely. We can eat just because it feels good. And lots of times we do.

**What are generations?** They're the groups of people who were born at around the same time. You and your brothers and sisters and cousins are in one generation, while your parents and aunts and uncles are in another generation, and your grandparents and their brothers and sisters are in a third generation, and so on.

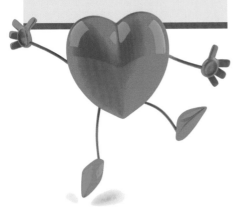

Meanwhile, our bodies are doing what they're supposed to, storing the energy from our food in the form of fat—but that fat never gets used. It just keeps on being stored, while we get heavier and heavier.

Gene aren't the whole story, though. If they were, the world would have had a bigger obesity problem for a longer time. Instead, the obesity problem has been growing worse and worse only over the past forty years.

Other things besides genes influence whether or not you're overweight. Environment—the people and things around you, the way you live—is the other piece of the story. Your family's lifestyle shapes how you act, how you grow, and how you will live even when you're a grownup and out on your own.

**What are traditions?**
They're the things we do and the way we do them that are special to a group we belong to, like our family or a group of friends. Usually, traditions have to do with what we do, how we do it, and when we do it.

# FAMILY LIFESTYLE AND OBESITY

No two families are exactly alike. Some things about your family's lifestyle are special and like no other. For example, maybe your family has a special meal they eat to celebrate birthdays. Or maybe your grandmother always makes a certain kind of cookie whenever you go to her house. Maybe your family always goes biking together on Saturdays. Or instead, maybe you spend your weekends curled up reading and watching television.

Family **traditions** are different from one household to another. So if your family loves

*Start family traditions that do not center around eating or sitting in front of the television. Get outside with your family and play games or go hiking!*

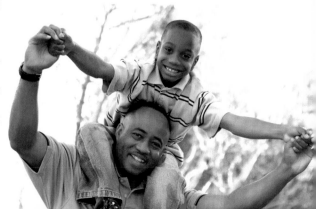

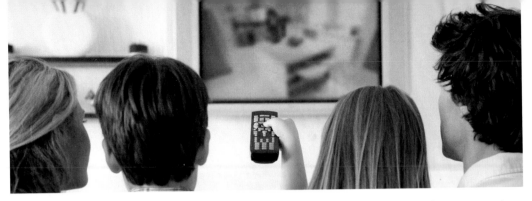

*Spending time with your family is important, but watching too much T.V. together is not the healthiest lifestyle choice for any of you.*

to exercise together, you're more likely to burn off the calories you eat—and less likely to be overweight. But if your family likes to do only sitting-down activities, then you may never have learned that exercise can be fun—and your body may have a harder time burning off the calories you eat. Now suppose your family loves to sit around the living room watching television and eating cookies and ice cream. Or maybe you have huge "Sunday dinners" every night at your house. Your family loves to eat together, they seldom exercise—and chances are good that you (and the other members of your family) are likely to be overweight.

**What does unique mean?** It means one-of-a-kind. If something is unique, there's nothing else exactly like it in the whole world.

But even though every family is **unique**, some things about your family's lifestyle probably aren't all that different from other families'. The world around your family shapes how they behave as well—and the world has changed in the past forty years or so.

For one thing, serving sizes have become larger. A group of doctors studied five kinds of food—hamburgers, Mexican food, soft drinks, snacks, and pizza—and found that serving sizes for all of them except pizza had gotten bigger since 1971. Hamburgers today are one-fifth bigger than they were in 1971. A plate of Mexican food is usually one-quarter bigger. In 1971, most soft drinks were 12 ounces, but today, many are 20 ounces—and they come with free refills. And serving sizes for snack foods like potato chips and pretzels are two-thirds bigger than they once

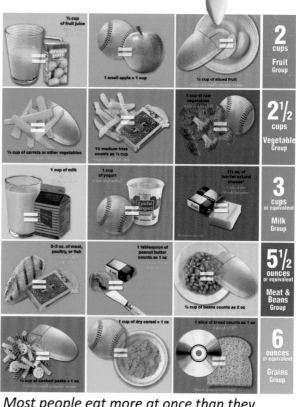

*Most people eat more at once than they should. This chart shows healthy portion sizes compared to the sizes of everyday objects like baseballs and computer mice.*

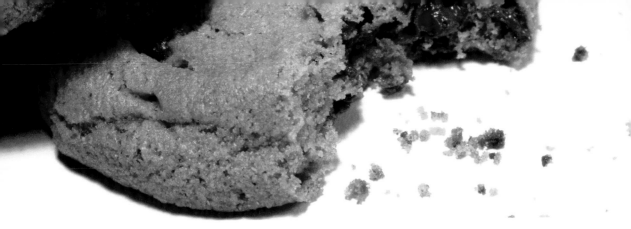

were! The doctors also discovered that it's not just at restaurants where serving sizes are bigger. People are eating bigger servings at home too.

Of course, just because you're given a lot of food, doesn't mean you have to eat it. But chances are you will! Even if you don't eat the whole thing, you'll at least you'll eat more than you would have if you'd been given a smaller serving.

Another group of doctors proved that this was true. They gave people two meals on two different days. Each meal was macaroni and cheese, but one time the doctors gave the people small servings and the other time they gave them big servings. Both times, the doctors told the people to eat until they were full. Not everyone cleaned his plate either time (even when the servings were small)—but even if he didn't finish all the macaroni he'd been given, everyone ate about one-third more when he had big servings than when he had small servings. And the people told the doctors they hadn't even noticed that the servings were different sizes!

So when we're given bigger servings everywhere we turn, it's no wonder we're gaining weight! But there's still more to the obesity story. It's not just how much we eat that's the problem. It's also WHAT we eat.

More and more people in the world today are eating foods made out of white flour and white sugar. Our bodies break down the energy in these foods very quickly and easily. These foods make more energy than our bodies can usually use all at once, so we store the energy as fat. But because white flour and white sugar break down so quickly, we also tend to feel hungry sooner. So we eat MORE.

Where do we find white flour and white sugar? In cookies and cakes, in white bread and rolls, in prepackaged meals, in many snacks, in candy, in pasta that's not made from whole wheat, and in many fast foods. If your family is like most families, these foods are a part of your diet every day.

If you're used to eating these kinds of foods, they are probably the kinds of food you like best. They taste good to you. So you're likely to fill up on them instead of

*The more you eat veggies, the more you will learn to like them.*

eating things like vegetables, fruit, and whole-grain foods. Be honest—if you had to choose, would you pick a bowl of ice cream or a bowl of broccoli? But you might be surprised to find that the more often you eat vegetables, the more you'll like them. We tend to like what we're used to—and this means we can change our tastes.

But there's still one more important thing in the lifestyle chapter of the obesity story—and that's exercise. If we were eating more calories but exercising more, we wouldn't have such a big problem. But instead, we're doing just the opposite—we're eating more and exercising less.

Even fifty years ago, most grownups had plenty of physical work to do that kept them active. Keeping a house clean and growing food took up a lot of time—and burned a lot of calories. Children had chores to do, as well, and when their chores were done, they played games like tag and hide-and-go-seek and hopscotch. All these games involved MOVING. In those days, people moved their bodies every single day.

But that's not the way we live today. Laborsaving inventions like washing machines and vacuum cleaners mean we can keep our homes and clothing clean without working so hard. We buy our food at the grocery store, and often it comes in quick, easy-to-fix packages—or we eat out at a restaurant. Daily life just doesn't take as much effort as it once did.

That seems like a good thing. After all, if we have less work to do, then we have more time to enjoy ourselves. And that

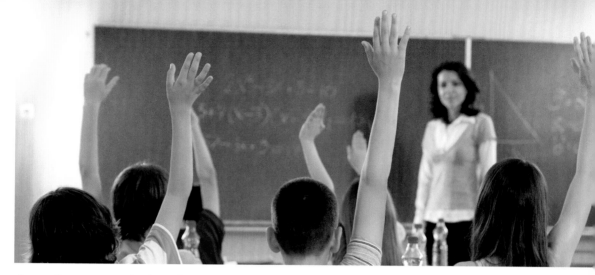

*According to a study done by the University of Michigan, children spend 32.5 hours a week in school, more than 14 hours a week watching T.V., and about 3 hours a week using home computers. This adds up to almost 50 hours a week of sitting!*

would be fine too—except the things we do today to enjoy ourselves often don't involve moving our bodies.

Think about what most people do every day. Many grown-ups work in an office where they sit in front of a computer all day. Children go to school, where for much of the day they sit at desks. In the evenings, families come home from school and from work—and then what do they do? Chances are, they sit down and watch television. They might listen to music on their iPods or MP3 players. Or they sit at their computers and play games or surf the Net.

And then they go to bed, get up the next morning—and spend another day sitting. No wonder so many adults and children are obese or overweight!

If genetics and lifestyle are working against so many people, what can they do? Should they just give up and be over-weight?

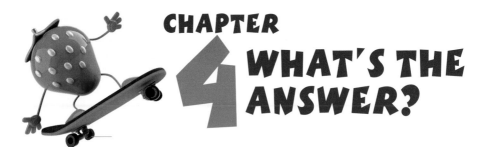

# CHAPTER 4
# WHAT'S THE ANSWER?

Obesity doesn't have any easy answers—not for the world as a whole, and not for individuals. If you or someone you know is overweight or obese, you probably already know how hard it is to lose weight and keep it off. No one should ever be blamed for being overweight. It's a very, very difficult problem.

Scientists and doctors are working together to find the cure for this serious health problem—but they haven't found it yet.

So in the meantime, what can we do? We can't change our family traditions all at once. We can do even less about the life-style that an entire society is living all around us. And we can't do anything at all about the genes we inherited from our parents!

## DID YOU KNOW?

Researchers have found that going on a special diet is not usually the best way to lose weight. Diets are just too hard to stick to.

# THE FIRST STEP: GET EDUCATED!

The first thing you as an individual can do is to be aware of the problem. Talk about it with your family and friends. The more people know about a problem and the more they think about it and talk about it, the more families and societies begin to change, little by little.

Don't just accept what goes on around you and follow along blindly. Ask questions. Learn about what a healthy lifestyle looks like. Find out about healthier ways to eat. Discover for yourself how exercise helps your body be the best it can be.

Eating a variety of foods is the best way to get all the things your body needs to be healthy. Whole or unprocessed foods—foods that are as close as possible to the way they grew naturally, without being frozen, canned, or packaged—are the best choices for getting what your body needs.

Does this mean you have to give up foods like potato chips, candy bars, and cookies forever? No, it's okay to have these foods once in a while. Just don't eat too many of them. To choose healthier foods, check food labels, and then pick foods that are high in vitamins and minerals. For example, if you're choosing a drink, a glass of milk is a **nutritious** choice—but a glass of

**What does nutritious mean?** Something that's nutritious is a food or drink that provides your body with the tools it needs to stay healthy.

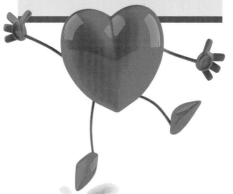

soda doesn't give you much nutrition, if any, but it does have lots of lots of calories!

# THE SECOND STEP: TAKE AN HONEST LOOK AT YOURSELF!

You may not be overweight or obese now. But as you get older, you might gain weight, depending on your genes and your lifestyle. To find out if you're likely to have a problem with your weight as you get older, answer the following questions as honestly as you can:

1. Do you usually take less than twenty minutes to eat a meal?
2. After finishing your meal, do you still feel hungry?
3. When you sit down to eat, do you eat everything put in front of you no matter how big the portion size?
4. Does your diet include large amounts of high-sugar or high-fat foods?
5. Do you exercise at least three days each week?
6. Do you eat a balanced diet each and every day?

## DID YOU KNOW?

Scientists have discovered the best combination of foods your body needs to be healthy. A diagram of this combination looks like a pyramid, with the foods you need to eat more at the bottom, and the foods you need to eat less at the top. The U.S. Department of Agriculture, the part of the American government that deals with food, farming, and nutrition, has created a picture called "MyPyramid" to help you understand better how much and what kinds of foods you need to eat in order to be healthy.

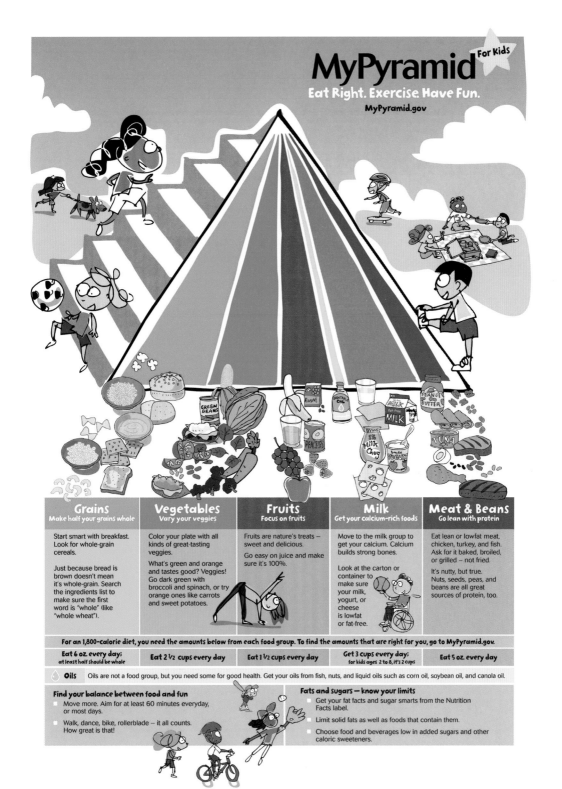

# MyPyramid For Kids
## Eat Right. Exercise. Have Fun.
### MyPyramid.gov

| **Grains** Make half your grains whole | **Vegetables** Vary your veggies | **Fruits** Focus on fruits | **Milk** Get your calcium-rich foods | **Meat & Beans** Go lean with protein |
|---|---|---|---|---|
| Start smart with breakfast. Look for whole-grain cereals. | Color your plate with all kinds of great-tasting veggies. | Fruits are nature's treats — sweet and delicious. | Move to the milk group to get your calcium. Calcium builds strong bones. | Eat lean or lowfat meat, chicken, turkey, and fish. Ask for it baked, broiled, or grilled – not fried. |
| Just because bread is brown doesn't mean it's whole-grain. Search the ingredients list to make sure the first word is "whole" (like "whole wheat"). | What's green and orange and tastes good? Veggies! Go dark green with broccoli and spinach, or try orange ones like carrots and sweet potatoes. | Go easy on juice and make sure it's 100%. | Look at the carton or container to make sure your milk, yogurt, or cheese is lowfat or fat-free. | It's nutty, but true. Nuts, seeds, peas, and beans are all great sources of protein, too. |

For an 1,800-calorie diet, you need the amounts below from each food group. To find the amounts that are right for you, go to MyPyramid.gov.

| Eat 6 oz. every day; at least half should be whole | Eat 2 ½ cups every day | Eat 1 ½ cups every day | Get 3 cups every day; for kids ages 2 to 8, it's 2 cups | Eat 5 oz. every day |
|---|---|---|---|---|

**◌ Oils**   Oils are not a food group, but you need some for good health. Get your oils from fish, nuts, and liquid oils such as corn oil, soybean oil, and canola oil.

### Find your balance between food and fun
- Move more. Aim for at least 60 minutes everyday, or most days.
- Walk, dance, bike, rollerblade – it all counts. How great is that!

### Fats and sugars — know your limits
- Get your fat facts and sugar smarts from the Nutrition Facts label.
- Limit solid fats as well as foods that contain them.
- Choose food and beverages low in added sugars and other caloric sweeteners.

If you answered yes to the first three questions or no to questions 5 and 6, you may find that you gain weight as you get older. But don't wait till you have a problem! The more weight you have to lose, the harder it is to do. Do what you can to change your life-style now.

# THE THIRD STEP: TAKE ACTION!

The best way to lose weight, experts tell us, is to change the way you live. Form new habits. This isn't easy—but new ways of living become easier to do the more we do them. Learn to take care of your body every day. Give it the foods it needs to be healthy. And then find fun ways to get more exercise, which will also help keep your body at the right weight.

## DID YOU KNOW?

Scientists have discovered the best combination of foods your body needs to be healthy. A diagram of this combination looks like a pyramid, with the foods you need to eat more at the bottom, and the foods you need to eat less at the top. The U.S. Department of Agriculture, the part of the American government that deals with food, farming, and nutrition, has created a picture called "MyPyramid" to help you understand better how much and what kinds of foods you need to eat in order to be healthy.

## DID YOU KNOW?

If you haven't been moving around much lately, start out slowly. Don't overdo it! It will be harder to stick with an exercise program if you make yourself tired and sore at the very beginning.

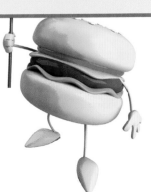

We're all in this together. Because of our heredity, some of us may have a bigger problem than others—but all of us live in a changing world where eating healthy and exercising have become harder to do. While scientists and doctors search for the answers to this problem, we can do what we can in our individual lives.

And just because you're still a kid doesn't mean you can't begin now. Get educated, be honest with yourself, and take action! No matter the genes and lifestyle you inherited from your family, no matter how hard it may be to change, you have the power to shape your life.

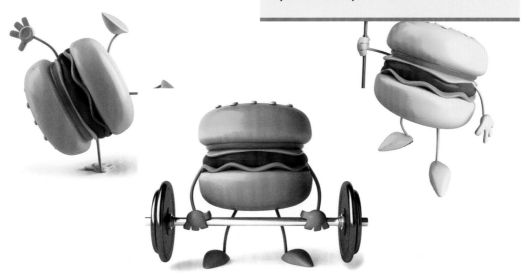

### DID YOU KNOW?

Exercise should be fun. So pick something you genuinely enjoy doing. You'll be more likely to make exercise a habit if you like what you're doing.

# READ MORE ABOUT IT

Bean, Anita. *Awesome Foods for Active Kids: The ABCs of Eating for Energy and Health*. Alameda, Calif.: Hunter House, 2006.

Behan, Eileen. *Fit Kids: Raising Physically and Emotionally Strong Kids with Real Food*. New York: Pocket Publishing, 2001.

Berg, Frances M. *Children and Teens Afraid to Eat*. Hettinger, N.D.: Healthy Weight Network, 2001.

Dolgoff, Joanna. *Red Light, Green Light, Eat Right: The Food Solution That Lets Kids Be Kids.* Emmaus, Penn.: Rodale, 2009.

Gaesser, Glenn. *Big Fat Lies: The Truth About Your Weight and Your Health.* Carlsbad, Calif.: Gürze Books, 2002.

Johnson, Susan and Laurel Mellin. *Just for Kids! (Obesity Prevention Workbook)*. San Anselmo, Calif.: Balboa Publishing, 2002.

Lillien, Lisa. *Hungry Girl 1-2-3: The Easiest, Most Delicious, Guilt-Free Recipes on the Planet*. New York: St. Martin's, 2010.

Vos, Miriam B. *The No-Diet Obesity Solution for Kids*. Bethesda, Md.: AGA Institute, 2009.

Wann, Marilyn. *Fat! So? Because You Don't Have to Apologize for Your Size*. Berkeley. Calif.: Ten Speed Press, 2009.

Zinczenko, David and Matt Goulding. *Eat This Not That! For Kids!* Emmaus, Penn.: Rodale, 2008.

# FIND OUT MORE ON THE INTERNET

About Our Kids: Obesity and Overweight
www.aboutourkids.org/aboutour/
articles/gr_obesity_03.html

Activity Cards
www.bam.gov/sub_physicalactivity/
physicalactivity_activitycards.html

Aim for a Healthy Weight: Assess
Your Risk
www.nhlbi.nih.gov/health/public/
heart/obesity/lose_wt/risk.
htm#limitations

American Obesity Association
www.obesity.org

Environmental Contributions to Obesity
www.endotext.org/obesity/obesity7/
obesity7.htm

The Learning Center
www.hebs.scot.nhs.uk/learningcentre/
obesity/intro/index.cfm

Obesity: Causes
www.weight-loss-i.com/obesity-causes.
htm

Obesity and Environment Factsheet
www.niehs.nih.gov/oc/factsheets/
obesity.htm

Move It!
www.fns.usda.gov/tn/tnrockyrun/
moveit.htm

MyPyramid Blast Off Game
www.mypyramid.gov/kids/kids_game.
html

Small Step Kids
www.smallstep.gov/kids/html/games_
and_activities.html

The websites listed on this page were active at the time of publication. The publisher is not responsible for websites that have changed their address or discontinued operation since the date of publication. The publisher will review and update the websites upon each reprint.

# INDEX

# PICTURE CREDITS

## ABOUT THE AUTHOR

Rae Simons has ghostwritten several adult books on dieting and obesity. She is also the author of more than thirty young adult books. She lives in upstate New York, where she tries hard to get enough exercise and eat healthy foods.

.